HYPOTHYROIDISM JUICING RECIPES COOKBOOK

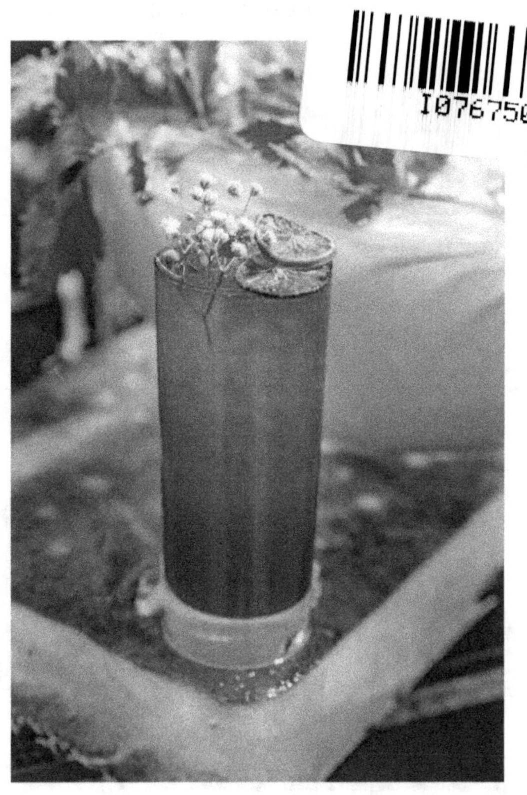

DR. JESSICA SMITH

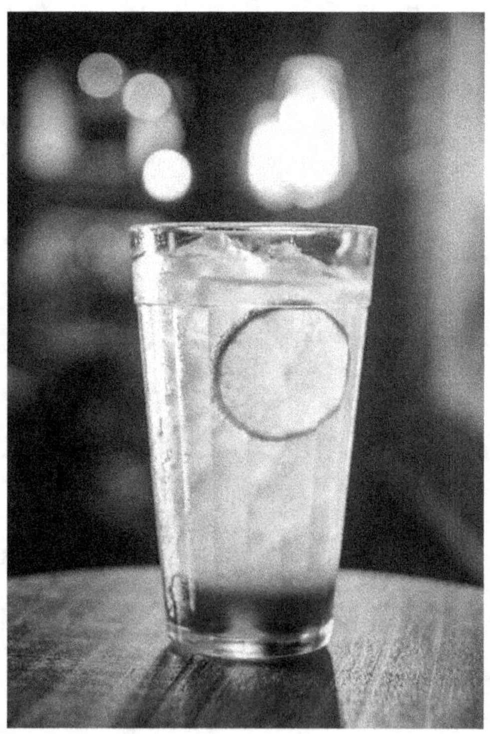

TABLE OF CONTENTS

HOW TO USE HYPOTHYROIDISM JUICING COOKBOOK

➢ **Introduction Familiarization:**

Begin by reading the introduction section of the cookbook. Gain insights into the purpose of the recipes, their impact on hypothyroidism, and the overall philosophy behind the culinary choices.

➢ **Understanding Hypothyroidism:**

Educate yourself about hypothyroidism and its dietary implications. Recognize the specific nutrients and ingredients that can support thyroid health. The cookbook may provide background information on how certain foods positively influence thyroid function.

➢ **Recipe Selection:**

Take time to browse through the juicing recipes. Identify those that align with your taste preferences, dietary restrictions, and ingredients available in your pantry. The cookbook likely offers a variety of options to suit different palates.

➢ **Gather Ingredients:**

Create a shopping list based on the recipes you've chosen. Ensure you have the necessary fruits, vegetables, and additional ingredients required for the juicing process. Fresh, high-quality produce is key to maximizing nutritional benefits.

> **Equipment Check:**

Confirm that you have the necessary kitchen tools, such as a quality juicer or blender, to effectively execute the recipes. Clean and prepare the equipment before starting the juicing process.

> **Follow Step-by-Step Instructions:**

Turn to the chosen recipe and carefully follow the step-by-step instructions. Pay attention to specific details such as ingredient quantities, order of blending, and recommended settings on your juicer or blender.

> **Experiment and Customize:**

Feel free to experiment with ingredient proportions based on personal taste preferences. If the cookbook encourages customization, use it as an opportunity to tailor the recipes to your liking while still adhering to the principles of hypothyroidism-friendly nutrition.

> **Incorporate into Daily Routine:**

Integrate the juicing recipes into your daily routine. Consider incorporating them as refreshing morning beverages, afternoon pick-me-ups, or even as part of your meals. Consistency is key to experiencing the potential benefits.

➢ **Monitor and Reflect:**

Pay attention to how your body responds to the hypothyroidism juicing recipes. Monitor energy levels, mood, and any changes in symptoms related to thyroid health. Keeping a journal can help you track progress and identify patterns.

➢ **Consult with Healthcare Professionals:**

While the cookbook may offer valuable insights, it's essential to consult with your healthcare provider or a registered dietitian. They can provide personalized advice based on your specific health condition, ensuring that the recipes complement your overall treatment plan.

By following these 10 steps, you can effectively use the Hypothyroidism Juicing Recipes Cookbook as a valuable resource in supporting your thyroid health through nutritious and delicious juices.

Understanding Hypothyroidism Disease

Hypothyroidism is a common endocrine disorder characterized by an underactive thyroid gland, leading to insufficient production of thyroid hormones—primarily thyroxine (T4) and triiodothyronine (T3).

The thyroid hormones play a crucial role in regulating the body's metabolism, energy production, and overall growth and development. When the thyroid gland fails to produce an adequate amount of hormones, it results in a slowing down of bodily functions.

Common symptoms of hypothyroidism include fatigue, weight gain, sensitivity to cold, dry skin, hair loss, and muscle weakness.

Due to its gradual onset and often subtle symptoms, hypothyroidism may go unnoticed or be attributed to other factors, making accurate diagnosis challenging.

The primary cause of hypothyroidism is often autoimmune thyroiditis, also known as Hashimoto's disease, where the immune system mistakenly attacks the thyroid tissue.

Other causes may include iodine deficiency, certain medications, radiation therapy, or congenital factors.

Diagnosis involves blood tests measuring thyroid hormone levels, specifically TSH (thyroid-stimulating hormone), T4, and T3. Treatment typically involves thyroid hormone replacement therapy to restore hormone levels and alleviate symptoms.

Managing hypothyroidism requires ongoing monitoring and adjustments to medication, emphasizing the importance of regular communication between individuals and healthcare professionals to optimize thyroid health and overall well-being.

Principles Of Hypothyroidism

The principles underlying hypothyroidism revolve around the dysfunction of the thyroid gland, a small butterfly-shaped organ in the neck responsible for producing essential hormones that regulate metabolism and various bodily functions.

When these principles are disrupted, hypothyroidism ensues.

The primary principle lies in the inadequate production of thyroid hormones, primarily thyroxine (T4) and triiodothyronine (T3). These hormones play a pivotal role in controlling energy expenditure, temperature regulation, and cellular metabolism. In hypothyroidism, the thyroid gland fails to generate a sufficient quantity of these hormones, leading to a slowing down of bodily processes.

Autoimmune thyroiditis, or Hashimoto's disease, represents a fundamental principle of hypothyroidism.

This condition occurs when the immune system erroneously attacks the thyroid tissue, impairing its ability to produce hormones. Other principles include iodine deficiency, a crucial component in thyroid hormone synthesis, certain medications, radiation therapy, or congenital factors.

Recognizing these principles is integral to understanding the varied and often subtle symptoms associated with hypothyroidism, such as fatigue, weight gain, and cognitive impairment. Diagnosis hinges on measuring thyroid hormone levels through blood tests, with treatment typically involving hormone replacement therapy.

Effectively managing hypothyroidism requires a comprehensive approach, addressing both the autoimmune and hormonal aspects. Principles of treatment involve restoring thyroid hormone balance, continuous monitoring, and individualized care to alleviate symptoms and improve overall well-being.

Benefits of Hypothyroidism Juicing

A Hypothyroidism Juicing Recipes Cookbook offers a wealth of benefits for individuals navigating the challenges of an underactive thyroid.

Firstly, these recipes are crafted with a keen understanding of the nutrients essential for thyroid health. Ingredients such as selenium, zinc, and iodine, crucial for thyroid function, are thoughtfully incorporated, potentially aiding in the optimization of hormonal balance.

The cookbook's recipes often feature fruits and vegetables rich in antioxidants, vitamins, and minerals, offering a nutritional boost that may support the immune system and help mitigate inflammation associated with autoimmune thyroid conditions like Hashimoto's disease.

The inclusion of ingredients with anti-inflammatory properties, such as ginger and turmeric, may contribute to reducing inflammation often linked to thyroid disorders.

Furthermore, the recipes emphasize a holistic approach to health, promoting whole, unprocessed foods that can positively impact weight management—a significant concern for individuals with hypothyroidism.

These juices may provide a convenient and delicious way to consume a variety of nutrients that support overall well-being, from enhancing energy levels to supporting skin health and improving digestion.

Ultimately, the benefits of a Hypothyroidism Juicing Recipes Cookbook extend beyond merely addressing nutritional needs; they offer a flavorful and accessible avenue for individuals to proactively engage in their well-being, fostering a sense of empowerment and promoting a positive relationship with food for those managing thyroid-related challenges.

Tips for Hypothyroidism Juicing

Navigating hypothyroidism with juicing involves thoughtful considerations to harness the nutritional benefits while aligning with the specific needs of an underactive thyroid.

Here are valuable tips for incorporating juicing into a hypothyroidism-friendly lifestyle:

➢ **Iodine-Rich Ingredients:**

Prioritize ingredients rich in iodine, a crucial component for thyroid hormone synthesis. Incorporate seaweed, sea vegetables, and iodized salt judiciously into your juices.

➢ **Selenium Boost:**

Choose ingredients high in selenium, an essential mineral for thyroid function. Brazil nuts, sunflower seeds, and spinach can be excellent additions.

➢ **Mindful Cruciferous Consumption:**

While cruciferous vegetables like broccoli and kale offer health benefits, consume them in moderation. Excessive intake may affect thyroid function, so rotate them with other greens.

➢ **Anti-Inflammatory Additions:**

Include anti-inflammatory ingredients like ginger and turmeric to potentially alleviate inflammation associated with autoimmune thyroid conditions such as Hashimoto's disease.

➢ **Balanced Nutrient Profile:**

Strive for a balanced nutrient profile in your juices, incorporating a mix of fruits, vegetables, and leafy greens to provide a spectrum of vitamins and minerals.

➢ **Hydration is Key:**

Stay adequately hydrated. Water-rich fruits and vegetables like cucumber and watermelon can contribute to hydration, supporting overall well-being.

➢ **Monitor Crucial Nutrients:**

Keep an eye on essential nutrients such as vitamin D, B vitamins, and iron. Juicing can be a supplementary source, but a well-rounded diet is vital for comprehensive nutrition.

➢ **Consult with Healthcare Professionals:**

Prior to making significant dietary changes, consult with your healthcare provider or a registered dietitian. They can provide personalized guidance based on your specific health condition and nutritional needs.

➢ **Limit Added Sugars**:

Be mindful of added sugars in your juices. Opt for naturally sweet fruits and consider small amounts of natural sweeteners like honey or maple syrup.

➢ **Listen to Your Body:**

Pay attention to how your body responds to different ingredients. If you notice any adverse effects, adjust your juicing recipes accordingly.

By incorporating these tips, individuals with hypothyroidism can leverage the potential benefits of juicing to support their thyroid health while enjoying flavorful and nutritious beverages.

Guidelines of Hypothyroidism Juicing

Guidelines for juicing with hypothyroidism revolve around selecting ingredients that support thyroid health while being mindful of potential sensitivities.

Here's a set of guidelines to ensure a nourishing and thyroid-friendly juicing experience:

➢ **Iodine Awareness:**

Prioritize ingredients rich in iodine, such as seaweed, sea vegetables, and iodized salt. Iodine is crucial for thyroid function and hormone synthesis.

➢ **Optimal Selenium Intake:**

Include selenium-rich foods like Brazil nuts, sunflower seeds, and spinach to support thyroid function and reduce oxidative stress.

➢ **Mindful Cruciferous Consumption:**

While cruciferous vegetables offer health benefits, consume them in moderation. Rotate kale, broccoli, and cauliflower with other greens to minimize any potential impact on thyroid function.

➢ **Anti-Inflammatory Choices:**

Integrate anti-inflammatory ingredients like ginger and turmeric to potentially alleviate inflammation associated with autoimmune thyroid conditions.

➢ **Balanced Nutrient Composition:**

Ensure a balanced mix of fruits, vegetables, and leafy greens in your juices. This provides a diverse array of vitamins, minerals, and antioxidants beneficial for overall health.

➢ **Hydration Emphasis:**

Stay well-hydrated with water-rich fruits and vegetables like cucumber and watermelon. Proper hydration supports bodily functions and aids digestion.

➢ **Supplementary Nutrient Monitoring:**

Be aware of essential nutrients such as vitamin D, B vitamins, and iron. Juicing can complement these nutrients, but a varied diet is crucial for comprehensive nutrition.

> **Limit Added Sugars:**

Minimize added sugars in your juices. Opt for naturally sweet fruits and consider small amounts of natural sweeteners like honey or maple syrup.

> **Consultation with Professionals:**

Before making significant dietary changes, consult with healthcare professionals or a registered dietitian. Personalized guidance ensures alignment with specific health conditions and nutritional needs.

> **Self-Monitoring and Adjustments:**

Pay attention to how your body responds to different ingredients. If any adverse effects or sensitivities are noticed, adjust your juicing recipes accordingly. Regular self-monitoring supports optimal well-being.

By adhering to these guidelines, individuals with hypothyroidism can create nourishing juices that align with their specific dietary needs

Causes of Hypothyroidism

Hypothyroidism, a condition marked by an underactive thyroid gland, can arise from various causes, each impacting the thyroid's ability to produce essential hormones.

The primary causes include:

> **Autoimmune Thyroiditis (Hashimoto's Disease):**

The leading cause of hypothyroidism involves the immune system mistakenly attacking the thyroid tissue. Over time, this immune response damages the thyroid, impeding its capacity to produce hormones.

> **Iodine Deficiency:**

Iodine is a vital component for thyroid hormone synthesis. In regions where iodine intake is insufficient, the thyroid struggles to produce an adequate amount of hormones, leading to hypothyroidism.

> **Medications and Treatments:**

Certain medications, such as lithium and amiodarone, may adversely affect thyroid function, inducing hypothyroidism. Radiation therapy for head and neck cancers can also impact thyroid activity.

> **Congenital Factors:**

Some individuals are born with a dysfunctional thyroid or absent thyroid gland, a condition known as congenital hypothyroidism. This requires early detection and lifelong hormone replacement therapy.

➤ **Pituitary Gland Dysfunction:**

The pituitary gland, which regulates thyroid hormone production, may malfunction, leading to decreased stimulation of the thyroid. This dysfunction, known as secondary or central hypothyroidism, results in inadequate hormone secretion.

➤ **Thyroid Surgery:**

Surgical removal of part or all of the thyroid gland, often performed to treat thyroid cancer or nodules, can result in decreased hormone production and subsequent hypothyroidism.

Understanding these diverse causes is crucial for accurate diagnosis and effective management of hypothyroidism.

Types of Hypothyroidism

Hypothyroidism manifests in various types, each with distinct origins and implications for thyroid function. The primary types include:

➤ **Primary Hypothyroidism:**

This is the most common type, arising from dysfunction within the thyroid gland itself. Autoimmune thyroiditis, known as Hashimoto's disease, is a prevalent cause, where the immune system mistakenly attacks the thyroid tissue, leading to reduced hormone production.

➢ **Secondary Hypothyroidism:**

In this type, dysfunction occurs at the level of the pituitary gland, which fails to produce sufficient thyroid-stimulating hormone (TSH). Without adequate TSH, the thyroid gland receives reduced stimulation to produce hormones, resulting in hypothyroidism.

➢ **Tertiary Hypothyroidism:**

Tertiary hypothyroidism stems from malfunctioning hypothalamus, the part of the brain that signals the pituitary gland to release TSH. Insufficient TSH release ultimately impacts the thyroid's hormone production.

➢ **Subclinical Hypothyroidism:**

Subclinical hypothyroidism is characterized by slightly elevated TSH levels, but with normal thyroid hormone levels. It often presents without noticeable symptoms, and the decision to treat is based on individual factors and risk assessments.

➢ **Congenital Hypothyroidism:**

Occurring from birth, congenital hypothyroidism results from genetic factors affecting thyroid development or function. Early detection through newborn screening is crucial, and lifelong thyroid hormone replacement is typically required.

> **Iatrogenic Hypothyroidism:**

This type is induced by medical intervention, often thyroid surgery or radioactive iodine therapy for hyperthyroidism or thyroid cancer. The deliberate reduction of thyroid tissue or function leads to a need for lifelong hormone replacement.

Symptoms of Hypothyroidism Disease

Hypothyroidism, characterized by an underactive thyroid gland, presents a spectrum of symptoms that can gradually manifest, often making early detection challenging. Common symptoms include:

> **Fatigue:**

Individuals with hypothyroidism often experience persistent fatigue, even after a full night's sleep, due to the slowed metabolic processes.

> **Weight Gain:**

Unexplained weight gain or difficulty in losing weight is a prevalent symptom. The slowed metabolism can contribute to changes in body weight.

> **Cold Sensitivity:**

Hypothyroidism can lead to heightened sensitivity to cold temperatures, as the diminished thyroid function affects the body's ability to regulate temperature.

- **Dry Skin and Hair**:

Dry, rough skin and brittle hair are common symptoms. The decreased production of thyroid hormones affects skin and hair health.

- **Muscle Weakness and Aches:**

Weakness and muscle aches are frequent, as the metabolic slowdown impacts the efficiency of energy production in the muscles.

- **Joint Pain:**

Individuals with hypothyroidism may experience stiffness and pain in the joints, contributing to discomfort and reduced mobility.

- **Constipation:**

Sluggish bowel movements and constipation are typical symptoms, as the digestive system slows down.

- **Depression and Cognitive Issues:**

Hypothyroidism can affect mood, leading to symptoms of depression. Cognitive functions may also be impaired, with difficulties in concentration and memory.

> **Menstrual Irregularities:**

Women may experience irregular menstrual cycles, heavier periods, or increased menstrual cramping.

> **Hoarse Voice and Swelling:**

A hoarse voice and swelling in the neck, known as goiter, may occur due to the thyroid gland's enlargement.

Risk Factors of Hypothyroidism

Hypothyroidism is influenced by various risk factors that can contribute to the development of this common endocrine disorder. Key risk factors include:

> **Age and Gender:**

The risk of hypothyroidism increases with age, particularly in individuals over 60. Women, especially those over 60, are more prone to hypothyroidism than men.

> **Family History:**

A family history of thyroid disorders, particularly autoimmune conditions like Hashimoto's disease, increases the likelihood of developing hypothyroidism. There is a genetic predisposition involved in many cases.

➢ **Autoimmune Diseases:**

Individuals with autoimmune disorders, such as rheumatoid arthritis or type 1 diabetes, have a higher risk of developing autoimmune thyroiditis, a common cause of hypothyroidism.

➢ **Previous Thyroid Issues:**

Individuals who have undergone thyroid surgery or received radioactive iodine treatment for hyperthyroidism or thyroid cancer may be at an increased risk of hypothyroidism.

➢ **Iodine Intake:**

In regions with low iodine levels, there is an increased risk of hypothyroidism due to inadequate iodine for thyroid hormone synthesis.

➢ **Radiation Exposure:**

Exposure to radiation, especially in the neck area, as seen in radiation therapy for head and neck cancers, increases the risk of hypothyroidism.

➢ **Certain Medications:**

Some medications, such as lithium and amiodarone, can affect thyroid function and elevate the risk of hypothyroidism.

> **Pregnancy and Postpartum:**

Women are more susceptible to thyroid disorders during and after pregnancy. Postpartum thyroiditis, an inflammation of the thyroid post-childbirth, can lead to hypothyroidism.

Awareness of these risk factors is crucial for early detection and proactive management of hypothyroidism. Regular monitoring and consultation with healthcare professionals can help mitigate risks and ensure timely intervention if necessary.

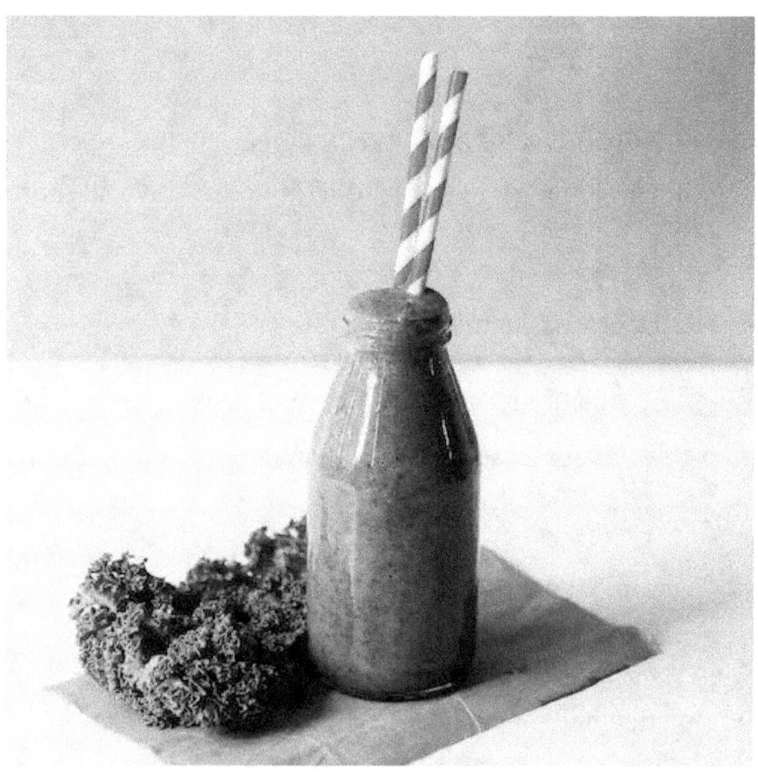

CHAPTER TWO

Breakfast Hypothyroidism Juicing Recipes

1. Berry Bliss Smoothie

Ingredients:

- ➢ 1 cup mixed berries (blueberries, raspberries, strawberries)
- ➢ 1/2 banana
- ➢ 1 tablespoon chia seeds
- ➢ 1 cup spinach leaves
- ➢ 1/2 cup coconut water

Instructions:

- ➢ Combine all ingredients in a blender.
- ➢ Blend until smooth.
- ➢ Pour into a glass and enjoy this antioxidant-rich smoothie.

Health Benefits:

- ➢ Berries provide antioxidants and vitamins.
- ➢ Banana adds natural sweetness and potassium.
- ➢ Chia seeds offer omega-3 fatty acids and additional fiber.
- ➢ Spinach provides iron and other essential nutrients.
- ➢ Coconut water adds hydration and a subtle tropical flavor.

Preparation Time: 5 minutes

2. Tropical Turmeric Elixir

Ingredients:

- ➢ 1 cup pineapple chunks
- ➢ 1/2 inch fresh ginger, peeled
- ➢ 1/2 teaspoon turmeric powder
- ➢ 1/2 cup Greek yogurt (or dairy-free alternative)
- ➢ 1 tablespoon honey
- ➢ 1 cup almond milk

Instructions:

- ➢ Blend pineapple, ginger, turmeric, Greek yogurt, honey, and almond milk until smooth.
- ➢ Pour into a glass.
- ➢ Revel in the tropical flavors of this anti-inflammatory elixir.

Health Benefits:

- ➢ Pineapple offers enzymes and vitamin C.
- ➢ Ginger and turmeric provide anti-inflammatory properties.
- ➢ Greek yogurt adds probiotics for gut health.
- ➢ Honey contributes natural sweetness with potential immune-boosting properties.
- ➢ Almond milk adds creaminess and calcium.

Preparation Time: 6 minutes

3. Green Energy Booster

Ingredients:

- ➤ 1 cucumber, peeled and chopped
- ➤ 1 green apple, cored and sliced
- ➤ 1 cup kale leaves
- ➤ 1/2 lemon, peeled
- ➤ 1 tablespoon flaxseeds
- ➤ 1 cup coconut water

Instructions:

- ➤ Blend cucumber, green apple, kale, lemon, flaxseeds, and coconut water until smooth.
- ➤ Pour into a glass.
- ➤ Savor the refreshing and nutrient-packed green goodness.

Health Benefits:

- ➤ Cucumber provides hydration and vitamins.
- ➤ Green apple adds natural sweetness and fiber.
- ➤ Kale offers a powerhouse of nutrients.
- ➤ Lemon contributes vitamin C and a zesty flavor.
- ➤ Flaxseeds provide omega-3 fatty acids and additional fiber.

Preparation Time: 7 minutes

4. Protein-Packed Almond Joy Shake

Ingredients:

- ➢ 1 cup almond milk
- ➢ 1/2 cup rolled oats
- ➢ 1 tablespoon almond butter
- ➢ 1 tablespoon cocoa powder
- ➢ 1/2 banana
- ➢ 1 teaspoon honey

Instructions:

- ➢ Blend almond milk, rolled oats, almond butter, cocoa powder, banana, and honey until smooth.
- ➢ Pour into a glass.
- ➢ Indulge in the rich and satisfying flavors of this protein-packed shake.

Health Benefits:

- ➢ Almond milk adds creaminess and calcium.
- ➢ Rolled oats provide complex carbohydrates and fiber.
- ➢ Almond butter contributes healthy fats and protein.
- ➢ Cocoa powder offers antioxidants and a chocolatey taste.
- ➢ Banana adds natural sweetness and potassium.

Preparation Time: 8 minutes

5. Citrus Sunrise Refresher

Ingredients:

- ➢ 2 oranges, peeled and segmented
- ➢ 1/2 grapefruit, peeled and segmented
- ➢ 1/2 lemon, peeled
- ➢ 1 tablespoon hemp seeds
- ➢ 1 cup coconut water

Instructions:

- ➢ Blend oranges, grapefruit, lemon, hemp seeds, and coconut water until smooth.
- ➢ Pour into a glass.
- ➢ Start your day with the invigorating flavors of this citrusy refresher.

Health Benefits:

- ➢ Oranges and grapefruit provide vitamin C and natural sweetness.
- ➢ Lemon adds a citrusy zing and more vitamin C.
- ➢ Hemp seeds offer omega-3 fatty acids and additional nutrients.
- ➢ Coconut water adds hydration and a mild tropical flavor.

Preparation Time: 5 minutes

6. Spinach and Pineapple Detox Blend

Ingredients:

- 2 cups fresh spinach leaves
- 1 cup pineapple chunks
- 1/2 cucumber, peeled and sliced
- 1/2 lime, peeled
- 1 tablespoon flaxseeds
- 1 cup coconut water

Instructions:

- Blend spinach, pineapple, cucumber, lime, flaxseeds, and coconut water until smooth.
- Pour into a glass.
- Enjoy this refreshing and detoxifying green blend.

Health Benefits:

- Spinach provides iron and essential nutrients.
- Pineapple offers enzymes and vitamin C.
- Cucumber adds hydration and vitamins.
- Lime contributes a citrusy twist and vitamin C.
- Flaxseeds provide omega-3 fatty acids and additional fiber.

Preparation Time: 6 minutes

7. Blueberry Banana Power Smoothie

Ingredients:

- ➢ 1 cup blueberries
- ➢ 1 banana
- ➢ 1/2 cup Greek yogurt (or dairy-free alternative)
- ➢ 1 tablespoon almond butter
- ➢ 1 teaspoon honey
- ➢ 1 cup almond milk

Instructions:

- ➢ Blend blueberries, banana, Greek yogurt, almond butter, honey, and almond milk until smooth.
- ➢ Pour into a glass.
- ➢ Recharge with the nutrient-rich goodness of this blueberry banana power smoothie.

Health Benefits:

- ➢ Blueberries offer antioxidants and vitamins.
- ➢ Banana adds natural sweetness and potassium.
- ➢ Greek yogurt provides probiotics for gut health.
- ➢ Almond butter contributes healthy fats and protein.
- ➢ Almond milk adds creaminess and calcium.

Preparation Time: 5 minutes

8. Carrot Cake Delight

Ingredients:

- ➤ 2 carrots, peeled and chopped
- ➤ 1/2 apple, cored and sliced
- ➤ 1/4 cup walnuts
- ➤ 1/2 teaspoon cinnamon
- ➤ 1 tablespoon chia seeds
- ➤ 1 cup coconut water

Instructions:

- ➤ Blend carrots, apple, walnuts, cinnamon, chia seeds, and coconut water until smooth.
- ➤ Pour into a glass.
- ➤ Savor the flavors reminiscent of carrot cake in this nutritious delight.

Health Benefits:

- ➤ Carrots provide beta-carotene and vitamins.
- ➤ Apple adds natural sweetness and fiber.
- ➤ Walnuts offer omega-3 fatty acids and additional nutrients.
- ➤ Cinnamon provides a warm and aromatic touch.
- ➤ Chia seeds contribute omega-3 fatty acids and additional fiber.

Preparation Time: 7 minutes

9. Avocado Berry Burst Smoothie

Ingredients:

- 1/2 avocado, peeled and pitted
- 1 cup mixed berries (strawberries, blueberries, raspberries)
- 1 tablespoon hemp seeds
- 1 tablespoon honey
- 1 cup almond milk

Instructions:

- Blend avocado, mixed berries, hemp seeds, honey, and almond milk until smooth.
- Pour into a glass.
- Delight in the creamy texture and vibrant flavors of this avocado berry burst.

Health Benefits:

- Avocado adds creaminess and healthy fats.
- Berries offer antioxidants and vitamins.
- Hemp seeds provide omega-3 fatty acids and additional nutrients.
- Honey contributes natural sweetness and potential immune-boosting properties.
- Almond milk adds a nutty flavor and calcium.

Preparation Time: 6 minutes

10. Quinoa and Mango Morning Refresher

Ingredients:

- 1/4 cup cooked quinoa, cooled
- 1/2 mango, peeled and diced
- 1/2 cup Greek yogurt (or dairy-free alternative)
- 1 tablespoon chia seeds
- 1 teaspoon honey
- 1 cup coconut water

Instructions:

- Blend cooked quinoa, mango, Greek yogurt, chia seeds, honey, and coconut water until smooth.
- Pour into a glass.
- Enjoy the unique combination of quinoa and mango in this morning refresher.

Health Benefits:

- Quinoa adds protein and fiber.
- Mango provides vitamins and natural sweetness.
- Greek yogurt offers probiotics for gut health.
- Chia seeds contribute omega-3 fatty acids and additional fiber.
- Coconut water adds hydration and a mild tropical flavor.

Preparation Time: 8 minutes

1. Green Goddess Gazpacho

Ingredients:

- ➢ 2 cucumbers, peeled and chopped
- ➢ 2 green bell peppers, seeded and chopped
- ➢ 2 celery stalks, chopped
- ➢ 1 cup spinach leaves
- ➢ 1/4 cup fresh parsley
- ➢ 1/2 lemon, peeled
- ➢ 2 tablespoons olive oil
- ➢ 1 teaspoon sea salt
- ➢ 1/2 teaspoon black pepper
- ➢ 1 cup coconut water

Instructions:

- ➢ Blend cucumbers, bell peppers, celery, spinach, parsley, lemon, olive oil, sea salt, black pepper, and coconut water until smooth.
- ➢ Chill in the refrigerator for at least 1 hour before serving.
- ➢ Serve in a bowl, and garnish with additional parsley if desired.

Health Benefits:

- ➢ Cucumbers provide hydration and vitamins.

- ➤ Bell peppers offer antioxidants and vitamin C.

- ➤ Spinach adds iron and essential nutrients.

- ➤ Lemon contributes a citrusy zing and vitamin C.

- ➤ Olive oil provides healthy fats and a smooth texture.

Preparation Time: 10 minutes

2. Quinoa and Vegetable Fusion

Ingredients:

- ➤ 1/2 cup cooked quinoa, cooled

- ➤ 1 carrot, peeled and chopped

- ➤ 1/2 beet, peeled and diced

- ➤ 1/2 cucumber, peeled and sliced

- ➤ 1/4 cup fresh cilantro

- ➤ 1/2 lime, peeled

- ➤ 1 tablespoon flaxseeds

- ➤ 1 cup coconut water

Instructions:

- ➤ Blend cooked quinoa, carrot, beet, cucumber, cilantro, lime, flaxseeds, and coconut water until smooth.

- ➤ Pour into a glass.

- ➤ Enjoy this nutrient-packed quinoa and vegetable fusion.

Health Benefits:

- ➤ Quinoa adds protein and fiber.

- ➢ Carrot and beet provide vitamins and antioxidants.
- ➢ Cucumber adds hydration and vitamins.
- ➢ Lime contributes a citrusy zing and vitamin C.
- ➢ Flaxseeds offer omega-3 fatty acids and additional fiber.

Preparation Time: 8 minutes

3. Sweet Potato and Turmeric Elixir

Ingredients:

- ➢ 1 sweet potato, cooked and cooled
- ➢ 1/2-inch fresh ginger, peeled
- ➢ 1/2 teaspoon turmeric powder
- ➢ 1/2 teaspoon cinnamon
- ➢ 1 tablespoon hemp seeds
- ➢ 1 cup almond milk

Instructions:

- ➢ Blend sweet potato, ginger, turmeric, cinnamon, hemp seeds, and almond milk until smooth.
- ➢ Pour into a glass.
- ➢ Savor the warmth and nutritional benefits of this sweet potato and turmeric elixir.

Health Benefits:

- ➢ Sweet potato provides vitamins and fiber.
- ➢ Ginger and turmeric offer anti-inflammatory properties.

- ➢ Cinnamon adds a warm and aromatic touch.
- ➢ Hemp seeds contribute omega-3 fatty acids and additional nutrients.
- ➢ Almond milk provides creaminess and calcium.

Preparation Time: 7 minutes

4. Mediterranean Greens Delight

Ingredients:

- ➢ 1 cup kale leaves
- ➢ 1/2 cucumber, peeled and sliced
- ➢ 1/4 cup olives (green or black)
- ➢ 1/2 cup cherry tomatoes
- ➢ 1/4 cup feta cheese (optional)
- ➢ 1/4 cup fresh basil leaves
- ➢ 1/2 lemon, peeled
- ➢ 2 tablespoons olive oil
- ➢ 1 teaspoon dried oregano
- ➢ 1 cup coconut water

Instructions:

- ➢ Blend kale, cucumber, olives, cherry tomatoes, feta cheese, basil, lemon, olive oil, dried oregano, and coconut water until smooth.
- ➢ Pour into a glass.

➤ Relish the flavors of the Mediterranean with this greens delight.

Health Benefits:

➤ Kale offers a powerhouse of nutrients.
➤ Cucumber provides hydration and vitamins.
➤ Olives contribute healthy fats and antioxidants.
➤ Cherry tomatoes add vitamins and a burst of flavor.
➤ Olive oil provides healthy fats and a smooth texture.

Preparation Time: 9 minutes

5. Protein-Packed Lentil Bliss

Ingredients:

➤ 1/2 cup cooked lentils, cooled
➤ 1 carrot, peeled and chopped
➤ 1/2 red bell pepper, seeded and chopped
➤ 1/4 cup red onion, chopped
➤ 1/4 cup fresh parsley
➤ 1/2 lemon, peeled
➤ 2 tablespoons olive oil
➤ 1 teaspoon cumin powder
➤ 1 cup vegetable broth

Instructions:

- Blend cooked lentils, carrot, red bell pepper, red onion, parsley, lemon, olive oil, cumin powder, and vegetable broth until smooth.
- Pour into a glass.
- Enjoy the protein-packed goodness of this lentil bliss.

Health Benefits:

- Lentils provide plant-based protein and fiber.
- Carrot and red bell pepper offer vitamins and antioxidants.
- Red onion adds flavor and potential anti-inflammatory properties.
- Lemon contributes a citrusy zing and vitamin C.
- Olive oil provides healthy fats and a smooth texture.

Preparation Time: 8 minutes

6. Chickpea and Spinach Power Blend

Ingredients:

- 1/2 cup cooked chickpeas, cooled
- 1 cup spinach leaves
- 1/2 cucumber, peeled and sliced
- 1/4 cup cherry tomatoes
- 1/4 cup red bell pepper, chopped
- 1/4 cup feta cheese (optional)

- ➢ 1/2 lemon, peeled
- ➢ 2 tablespoons olive oil
- ➢ 1 teaspoon dried oregano
- ➢ 1 cup coconut water

Instructions:

- ➢ Blend chickpeas, spinach, cucumber, cherry tomatoes, red bell pepper, feta cheese, lemon, olive oil, dried oregano, and coconut water until smooth.
- ➢ Pour into a glass.
- ➢ Experience the protein-packed goodness of this chickpea and spinach power blend.

Health Benefits:

- ➢ Chickpeas provide plant-based protein and fiber.
- ➢ Spinach offers iron and essential nutrients.
- ➢ Cucumber provides hydration and vitamins.
- ➢ Feta cheese adds a creamy texture and potential calcium.
- ➢ Olive oil contributes healthy fats and a smooth texture.

Preparation Time: 9 minutes

7. Broccoli and Avocado Elegance

Ingredients:

- ➢ 1 cup broccoli florets, steamed and cooled
- ➢ 1/2 avocado, peeled and pitted

- ➢ 1/2 cucumber, peeled and sliced
- ➢ 1/4 cup Greek yogurt (or dairy-free alternative)
- ➢ 1 tablespoon chia seeds
- ➢ 1/2 lime, peeled
- ➢ 1 cup coconut water

Instructions:

- ➢ Blend broccoli, avocado, cucumber, Greek yogurt, chia seeds, lime, and coconut water until smooth.
- ➢ Pour into a glass.
- ➢ Indulge in the elegance of this broccoli and avocado fusion.

Health Benefits:

- ➢ Broccoli provides vitamins and antioxidants.
- ➢ Avocado adds creamy texture and healthy fats.
- ➢ Cucumber provides hydration and vitamins.
- ➢ Greek yogurt offers probiotics for gut health.
- ➢ Chia seeds contribute omega-3 fatty acids and additional fiber.

Preparation Time: 7 minutes

8. Red Lentil and Tomato Harmony

Ingredients:

- ➢ 1/2 cup cooked red lentils, cooled
- ➢ 1 cup tomatoes, diced

- ➢ 1/2 red onion, chopped
- ➢ 1/4 cup fresh cilantro
- ➢ 1/2 lemon, peeled
- ➢ 2 tablespoons olive oil
- ➢ 1 teaspoon cumin powder
- ➢ 1/2 teaspoon paprika
- ➢ 1 cup vegetable broth

Instructions:

- ➢ Blend red lentils, tomatoes, red onion, cilantro, lemon, olive oil, cumin powder, paprika, and vegetable broth until smooth.
- ➢ Pour into a glass.
- ➢ Revel in the harmonious flavors of this red lentil and tomato blend.

Health Benefits:

- ➢ Red lentils provide plant-based protein and fiber.
- ➢ Tomatoes offer vitamins and antioxidants.
- ➢ Red onion adds flavor and potential anti-inflammatory properties.
- ➢ Lemon contributes a citrusy zing and vitamin C.
- ➢ Olive oil provides healthy fats and a smooth texture.

Preparation Time: 8 minutes

9. Zucchini and Basil Infusion

Ingredients:

- 1 zucchini, sliced
- 1/2 cup cherry tomatoes
- 1/4 cup fresh basil leaves
- 1/4 cup feta cheese (optional)
- 1/2 lemon, peeled
- 2 tablespoons olive oil
- 1/2 teaspoon garlic powder
- 1 cup vegetable broth

Instructions:

- Blend zucchini, cherry tomatoes, basil, feta cheese, lemon, olive oil, garlic powder, and vegetable broth until smooth.
- Pour into a glass.
- Enjoy the refreshing infusion of zucchini and basil.

Health Benefits:

- Zucchini provides vitamins and minerals.
- Cherry tomatoes offer vitamins and antioxidants.
- Basil adds flavor and potential anti-inflammatory properties.
- Feta cheese adds creaminess and potential calcium.
- Olive oil contributes healthy fats and a smooth texture.

Preparation Time: 7 minutes

10. Spicy Kale and Pineapple Kick

Ingredients:

- 1 cup kale leaves
- 1/2 cup pineapple chunks
- 1/2 cucumber, peeled and sliced
- 1/4 cup red bell pepper, chopped
- 1/4 teaspoon cayenne pepper (adjust to taste)
- 1/2 lime, peeled
- 2 tablespoons olive oil
- 1 cup coconut water

Instructions:

- Blend kale, pineapple, cucumber, red bell pepper, cayenne pepper, lime, olive oil, and coconut water until smooth.
- Pour into a glass.
- Savor the spicy kick of this kale and pineapple blend.

Health Benefits:

- Kale offers a powerhouse of nutrients.
- Pineapple provides enzymes and vitamin C.
- Cucumber provides hydration and vitamins.
- Red bell pepper adds flavor and antioxidants.
- Olive oil contributes healthy fats and a smooth texture.

Preparation Time: 8 minutes

1. Tomato Basil Bliss Soup

Ingredients:

- ➢ 2 cups tomatoes, diced
- ➢ 1/2 cup carrots, peeled and chopped
- ➢ 1/4 cup red bell pepper, chopped
- ➢ 1/4 cup fresh basil leaves
- ➢ 1/2 cup cooked quinoa, cooled
- ➢ 1/2 teaspoon garlic powder
- ➢ 1/2 teaspoon onion powder
- ➢ 1/2 teaspoon dried oregano
- ➢ 1 cup vegetable broth

Instructions:

- ➢ Blend tomatoes, carrots, red bell pepper, basil, quinoa, garlic powder, onion powder, dried oregano, and vegetable broth until smooth.
- ➢ Heat the mixture on the stovetop until warmed through.
- ➢ Serve in a bowl, garnished with additional fresh basil if desired.

Health Benefits:

- ➢ Tomatoes offer vitamins and antioxidants.
- ➢ Carrots provide beta-carotene and vitamins.

- ➤ Basil adds flavor and potential anti-inflammatory properties.

- ➤ Quinoa adds protein and fiber.

- ➤ Vegetable broth contributes essential nutrients.

Preparation Time: 12 minutes

2. Butternut Squash and Sage Elegance

Ingredients:

- ➤ 1 cup butternut squash, cooked and cooled

- ➤ 1/2 apple, cored and sliced

- ➤ 1/4 cup red onion, chopped

- ➤ 1 tablespoon fresh sage leaves

- ➤ 1/2 teaspoon cinnamon

- ➤ 1 tablespoon hemp seeds

- ➤ 1 cup almond milk

Instructions:

- ➤ Blend butternut squash, apple, red onion, sage, cinnamon, hemp seeds, and almond milk until smooth.

- ➤ Heat the mixture on the stovetop until warmed through.

- ➤ Savor the elegance of this butternut squash and sage creation.

Health Benefits:

- ➤ Butternut squash provides vitamins and antioxidants.

- ➤ Apple adds natural sweetness and fiber.

➢ Red onion offers flavor and potential anti-inflammatory properties.

➢ Sage adds a savory touch and potential digestive benefits.

➢ Almond milk provides creaminess and calcium.

Preparation Time: 10 minutes

3. Spinach and Lentil Nourishment Bowl

Ingredients:

➢ 1 cup cooked lentils, cooled

➢ 2 cups spinach leaves

➢ 1/2 cucumber, peeled and sliced

➢ 1/4 cup cherry tomatoes

➢ 1/4 cup feta cheese (optional)

➢ 1/2 lemon, peeled

➢ 2 tablespoons olive oil

➢ 1 teaspoon dried oregano

➢ 1 cup vegetable broth

Instructions:

➢ Blend cooked lentils, spinach, cucumber, cherry tomatoes, feta cheese, lemon, olive oil, dried oregano, and vegetable broth until smooth.

➢ Heat the mixture on the stovetop until warmed through.

➢ Serve in a bowl, garnished with additional feta if desired.

Health Benefits:

> Lentils provide plant-based protein and fiber.

> Spinach offers iron and essential nutrients.

> Cucumber provides hydration and vitamins.

> Feta cheese adds creaminess and potential calcium.

> Olive oil contributes healthy fats and a smooth texture.

Preparation Time: 11 minutes

4. Cauliflower and Broccoli Delight

Ingredients:

> 1 cup cauliflower florets, steamed and cooled

> 1 cup broccoli florets, steamed and cooled

> 1/2 avocado, peeled and pitted

> 1/4 cup fresh cilantro

> 1/2 lime, peeled

> 1 tablespoon chia seeds

> 1 cup coconut water

Instructions:

> Blend cauliflower, broccoli, avocado, cilantro, lime, chia seeds, and coconut water until smooth.

> Heat the mixture on the stovetop until warmed through.

> Enjoy the delightful combination of cauliflower and broccoli.

Health Benefits:

> ➤ Cauliflower and broccoli provide vitamins and antioxidants.
> ➤ Avocado adds creamy texture and healthy fats.
> ➤ Cilantro offers flavor and potential detoxification benefits.
> ➤ Lime contributes a citrusy zing and vitamin C.
> ➤ Chia seeds provide omega-3 fatty acids and additional fiber.

Preparation Time: 9 minutes

5. Turmeric Infused Carrot Harmony

Ingredients:

> ➤ 1 cup carrots, peeled and chopped
> ➤ 1/2 inch fresh ginger, peeled
> ➤ 1/2 teaspoon turmeric powder
> ➤ 1/2 teaspoon cumin powder
> ➤ 1/4 teaspoon black pepper
> ➤ 1 tablespoon hemp seeds
> ➤ 1 cup almond milk

Instructions:

> ➤ Blend carrots, ginger, turmeric, cumin, black pepper, hemp seeds, and almond milk until smooth.
> ➤ Heat the mixture on the stovetop until warmed through.
> ➤ Savor the harmonious flavors of this turmeric-infused carrot creation.

Health Benefits:

➢ Carrots provide beta-carotene and vitamins.

➢ Ginger and turmeric offer anti-inflammatory properties.

➢ Cumin adds a warm and aromatic touch.

➢ Hemp seeds provide omega-3 fatty acids and additional nutrients.

➢ Almond milk adds creaminess and calcium.

Preparation Time: 8 minutes

6. Green Bean and Almond Medley

Ingredients:

➢ 1 cup green beans, steamed and cooled

➢ 1/4 cup almonds

➢ 1/2 avocado, peeled and pitted

➢ 1/4 cup fresh parsley

➢ 1/2 lemon, peeled

➢ 2 tablespoons olive oil

➢ 1 teaspoon Dijon mustard

➢ 1 cup vegetable broth

Instructions:

➢ Blend green beans, almonds, avocado, parsley, lemon, olive oil, Dijon mustard, and vegetable broth until smooth.

➢ Heat the mixture on the stovetop until warmed through.

➤ Enjoy the medley of green beans and almonds in this nutritious blend.

Health Benefits:

➤ Green beans provide vitamins and minerals.
➤ Almonds offer healthy fats and additional nutrients.
➤ Avocado adds creaminess and healthy fats.
➤ Parsley provides flavor and potential detoxification benefits.
➤ Olive oil contributes healthy fats and a smooth texture.

Preparation Time: 10 minutes

7. Asparagus and Mushroom Delight

Ingredients:

➤ 1 cup asparagus, steamed and cooled
➤ 1/2 cup mushrooms, sliced
➤ 1/4 cup red onion, chopped
➤ 1/4 cup feta cheese (optional)
➤ 1/2 lemon, peeled
➤ 2 tablespoons olive oil
➤ 1 teaspoon dried thyme
➤ 1 cup vegetable broth

Instructions:

➤ Blend asparagus, mushrooms, red onion, feta cheese, lemon, olive oil, dried thyme, and vegetable broth until smooth.

- ➤ Heat the mixture on the stovetop until warmed through.
- ➤ Relish the delightful combination of asparagus and mushrooms.

Health Benefits:

- ➤ Asparagus provides vitamins and minerals.
- ➤ Mushrooms offer antioxidants and immune-boosting properties.
- ➤ Red onion adds flavor and potential anti-inflammatory benefits.
- ➤ Feta cheese adds creaminess and potential calcium.
- ➤ Olive oil contributes healthy fats and a smooth texture.

Preparation Time: 11 minutes

8. Cabbage and Apple Harvest

Ingredients:

- ➤ 1 cup cabbage, shredded
- ➤ 1/2 apple, cored and sliced
- ➤ 1/4 cup walnuts
- ➤ 1/4 cup fresh dill
- ➤ 1/2 lime, peeled
- ➤ 1 tablespoon hemp seeds
- ➤ 1 cup almond milk

Instructions:

> ➢ Blend cabbage, apple, walnuts, dill, lime, hemp seeds, and almond milk until smooth.
> ➢ Heat the mixture on the stovetop until warmed through.
> ➢ Enjoy the harvest flavors of this cabbage and apple fusion.

Health Benefits:

> ➢ Cabbage provides vitamins and fiber.
> ➢ Apples add natural sweetness and fiber.
> ➢ Walnuts offer omega-3 fatty acids and additional nutrients.
> ➢ Dill adds flavor and potential digestive benefits.
> ➢ Hemp seeds provide omega-3 fatty acids and additional fiber.

Preparation Time: 9 minutes

9. Eggplant and Tomato Symphony

Ingredients:

> ➢ 1 cup eggplant, roasted and cooled
> ➢ 1 cup tomatoes, diced
> ➢ 1/4 cup red bell pepper, chopped
> ➢ 1/4 cup fresh basil leaves
> ➢ 1/2 teaspoon garlic powder
> ➢ 1 tablespoon nutritional yeast (optional)
> ➢ 1 cup vegetable broth

Instructions:

> ➤ Blend eggplant, tomatoes, red bell pepper, basil, garlic powder, nutritional yeast, and vegetable broth until smooth.
> ➤ Heat the mixture on the stovetop until warmed through.
> ➤ Revel in the symphony of flavors in this eggplant and tomato blend.

Health Benefits:

> ➤ Eggplant provides vitamins and antioxidants.
> ➤ Tomatoes offer vitamins and immune-boosting properties.
> ➤ Basil adds flavor and potential anti-inflammatory benefits.
> ➤ Garlic powder contributes a savory touch and potential immune support.
> ➤ Nutritional yeast adds a cheesy flavor and potential B vitamins.

Preparation Time: 12 minutes

10. Bell Pepper and Quinoa Fiesta

Ingredients:

> ➤ 1 red bell pepper, chopped
> ➤ 1/2 cup cooked quinoa, cooled
> ➤ 1/4 cup black beans, cooked and cooled
> ➤ 1/4 cup corn kernels
> ➤ 1/4 cup fresh cilantro

- ➤ 1/2 lime, peeled
- ➤ 1 tablespoon olive oil
- ➤ 1 teaspoon cumin powder
- ➤ 1 cup vegetable broth

Instructions:

- ➤ Blend red bell pepper, quinoa, black beans, corn, cilantro, lime, olive oil, cumin powder, and vegetable broth until smooth.
- ➤ Heat the mixture on the stovetop until warmed through.
- ➤ Enjoy the fiesta of flavors in this bell pepper and quinoa concoction.

Health Benefits:

- ➤ Red bell pepper provides vitamins and antioxidants.
- ➤ Quinoa adds protein and fiber.
- ➤ Black beans offer plant-based protein and fiber.
- ➤ Corn contributes vitamins and minerals.
- ➤ Cilantro adds flavor and potential detoxification benefits.

Preparation Time: 10 minutes

Hypothyroidism Juicing Snacks Recipes

1. Avocado and Tomato Bruschetta

Ingredients:

➤ 1/2 avocado, mashed

➤ 1 cup cherry tomatoes, diced

➤ 1/4 cup red onion, finely chopped

➤ 1 tablespoon fresh basil, chopped

➤ 1/2 lemon, juiced

➤ Salt and pepper to taste

➤ Rice cakes or gluten-free crackers (optional)

Instructions:

➤ In a bowl, combine mashed avocado, diced tomatoes, red onion, and chopped basil.

➤ Squeeze fresh lemon juice over the mixture and season with salt and pepper to taste.

➤ Mix well and serve on rice cakes or gluten-free crackers.

Health Benefits:

➤ Avocado provides healthy fats and creamy texture.

➤ Tomatoes offer vitamins and antioxidants.

➤ Basil adds flavor and potential anti-inflammatory benefits.

➤ Lemon provides a citrusy zing and vitamin C.

Preparation Time: 10 minutes

2. Kale and Almond Pesto Dip

Ingredients:

➤ 2 cups kale leaves, stems removed

- ➢ 1/2 cup almonds, toasted
- ➢ 1/4 cup nutritional yeast
- ➢ 1/2 lemon, juiced
- ➢ 1 clove garlic
- ➢ 1/4 cup olive oil
- ➢ Salt and pepper to taste
- ➢ Sliced cucumber or carrot sticks for dipping

Instructions:

- ➢ In a food processor, blend kale, toasted almonds, nutritional yeast, lemon juice, garlic, and olive oil until smooth.
- ➢ Season with salt and pepper to taste.
- ➢ Serve as a dip with sliced cucumber or carrot sticks.

Health Benefits:

- ➢ Kale provides vitamins and minerals.
- ➢ Almonds offer healthy fats and additional nutrients.
- ➢ Nutritional yeast adds a cheesy flavor and potential B vitamins.
- ➢ Lemon provides a citrusy zing and vitamin C.

Preparation Time: 12 minutes

3. Coconut Chia Pudding with Berries

Ingredients:

- ➢ 1/4 cup chia seeds

- ➤ 1 cup coconut milk
- ➤ 1/2 teaspoon vanilla extract
- ➤ 1 tablespoon honey or maple syrup
- ➤ Mixed berries for topping

Instructions:

- ➤ In a bowl, mix chia seeds, coconut milk, vanilla extract, and sweetener.
- ➤ Stir well and refrigerate for at least 2 hours or until the mixture thickens.
- ➤ Top with mixed berries before serving.

Health Benefits:

- ➤ Chia seeds provide omega-3 fatty acids and additional fiber.
- ➤ Coconut milk offers healthy fats and a creamy texture.
- ➤ Berries provide antioxidants and vitamins.

Preparation Time: 5 minutes (plus chilling time)

4. Cucumber and Hummus Bites

Ingredients:

- ➤ 1 cucumber, sliced
- ➤ 1/2 cup hummus
- ➤ Cherry tomatoes, sliced olives, or fresh herbs for garnish

Instructions:

> ➤ Slice cucumber into rounds.

> ➤ Spoon a small dollop of hummus onto each cucumber round.

> ➤ Garnish with sliced cherry tomatoes, olives, or fresh herbs.

Health Benefits:

> ➤ Cucumber provides hydration and vitamins.

> ➤ Hummus offers plant-based protein and fiber.

> ➤ Tomatoes add vitamins and antioxidants.

Preparation Time: 8 minutes

5. Spinach and Artichoke Guacamole

Ingredients:

> ➤ 1 cup fresh spinach, chopped

> ➤ 1/2 cup artichoke hearts, drained and chopped

> ➤ 2 ripe avocados, mashed

> ➤ 1/4 cup red onion, finely chopped

> ➤ 1 clove garlic, minced

> ➤ 1/2 lime, juiced

> ➤ Salt and pepper to taste

> ➤ Whole grain tortilla chips or vegetable sticks for dipping

Instructions:

> In a bowl, combine chopped spinach, artichoke hearts, mashed avocados, red onion, minced garlic, and lime juice.
> Season with salt and pepper to taste and mix well.
> Serve with whole grain tortilla chips or vegetable sticks for dipping.

Health Benefits:

> Spinach offers iron and essential nutrients.
> Artichoke hearts provide fiber and antioxidants.
> Avocado adds healthy fats and creamy texture.
> Lime provides a citrusy zing and vitamin C.

Preparation Time: 10 minutes

6. Quinoa and Vegetable Stuffed Bell Peppers

Ingredients:

> 2 bell peppers, halved and seeds removed
> 1/2 cup cooked quinoa, cooled
> 1/4 cup black beans, rinsed and drained
> 1/4 cup corn kernels
> 1/4 cup salsa
> 1/4 teaspoon cumin
> 1/4 teaspoon chili powder
> Fresh cilantro for garnish

Instructions:

> In a bowl, mix cooked quinoa, black beans, corn, salsa, cumin, and chili powder.
> Spoon the mixture into halved bell peppers.
> Garnish with fresh cilantro and serve.

Health Benefits:

> Quinoa provides protein and fiber.
> Black beans offer plant-based protein and fiber.
> Bell peppers provide vitamins and antioxidants.
> Salsa adds flavor with potential health benefits.

Preparation Time: 15 minutes

7. Greek Yogurt Parfait with Berries

Ingredients:

> 1 cup Greek yogurt (or dairy-free alternative)
> 1/4 cup granola
> Mixed berries (blueberries, strawberries, raspberries)
> 1 tablespoon honey or maple syrup (optional)

Instructions:

> In a glass, layer Greek yogurt, granola, and mixed berries.
> Repeat the layers until the glass is filled.
> Drizzle honey or maple syrup on top if desired.

Health Benefits:

> Greek yogurt provides probiotics for gut health.
> Granola offers fiber and additional nutrients.
> Berries provide antioxidants and vitamins.
> Preparation Time: 5 minutes

8. Sweet Potato and Cinnamon Bites

Ingredients:

> 1 sweet potato, cooked and sliced
> 1 tablespoon coconut oil, melted
> 1/2 teaspoon cinnamon
> 1 tablespoon almond butter (or nut butter of choice)
> Chopped nuts for garnish

Instructions:

> Preheat the oven to 400°F (200°C).
> Toss sweet potato slices in melted coconut oil and sprinkle with cinnamon.
> Roast in the oven for 15-20 minutes until golden.
> Drizzle almond butter on top and garnish with chopped nuts.

Health Benefits:

> Sweet potatoes offer vitamins and fiber.
> Coconut oil provides healthy fats.
> Cinnamon adds a warm and aromatic touch.

➢ Almond butter adds healthy fats and protein.

Preparation Time: 25 minutes

9. Edamame and Sea Salt Snack Bowl

Ingredients:

➢ 1 cup edamame, steamed and cooled

➢ Sea salt to taste

➢ Squeeze of fresh lemon juice

➢ Red pepper flakes for a kick (optional)

Instructions:

➢ In a bowl, toss steamed edamame with sea salt.

➢ Squeeze fresh lemon juice over the edamame.

➢ Sprinkle red pepper flakes for a spicy kick if desired.

Health Benefits:

➢ Edamame provides plant-based protein and fiber.

➢ Sea salt adds minerals in moderation.

➢ Lemon juice offers a citrusy zing and vitamin C.

Preparation Time: 8 minutes

10. Almond and Dark Chocolate Energy Bites

Ingredients:

➢ 1 cup almonds, finely chopped

- ➢ 1/4 cup dark chocolate chips
- ➢ 2 tablespoons honey or maple syrup
- ➢ 1/2 teaspoon vanilla extract
- ➢ Pinch of sea salt

Instructions:

- ➢ In a bowl, mix chopped almonds, dark chocolate chips, honey or maple syrup, vanilla extract, and a pinch of sea salt.
- ➢ Form the mixture into bite-sized balls.
- ➢ Chill in the refrigerator for at least 30 minutes before serving.

Health Benefits:

- ➢ Almonds provide healthy fats and protein.
- ➢ Dark chocolate offers antioxidants.
- ➢ Honey or maple syrup adds natural sweetness.
- ➢ Vanilla extract adds flavor without added calories.

Preparation Time: 15 minutes

CONCLUSION

Embarking on a journey towards better health through a hypothyroidism juicing recipes cookbook is not just a culinary experience but a commitment to nourishing your body and mind.

As we close the chapters of this cookbook, let's reflect on the powerful impact that thoughtful nutrition can have on managing hypothyroidism and fostering overall well-being.

These recipes aren't just a collection of ingredients and instructions; they are a manifestation of the understanding that each meal can be a step towards reclaiming control over your health.

The carefully crafted combinations of fruits, vegetables, and superfoods serve as a testament to the idea that holistic well-being starts in the kitchen.

From refreshing breakfast juices to satisfying dinner blends, each recipe encapsulates the principles of balance, nourishment, and flavor.

As you explore the diverse and delicious options presented within these pages, may you discover the joy of creating meals that not only support thyroid health but also awaken your taste buds to the vibrant spectrum of natural flavors.

Remember, this cookbook is a guide, an invitation to embrace a lifestyle that celebrates health and vitality. Let it be a constant companion on your journey, empowering you to make informed and delicious choices that resonate with your body's needs.

As you savor the wholesome goodness within these recipes, may you find inspiration to create a life filled with vitality, wellness, and the satisfaction of sipping on the elixir of well-being. Here's to your health, happiness, and the flavorful chapters that lie ahead!